WHIPLASH: More Than Just Neck Pain

An overview of why you may hurt all over and what symptoms to watch out for after physical trauma.

DR. KARIN DRUMMOND

WHIPLASH:
More Than Just Neck Pain

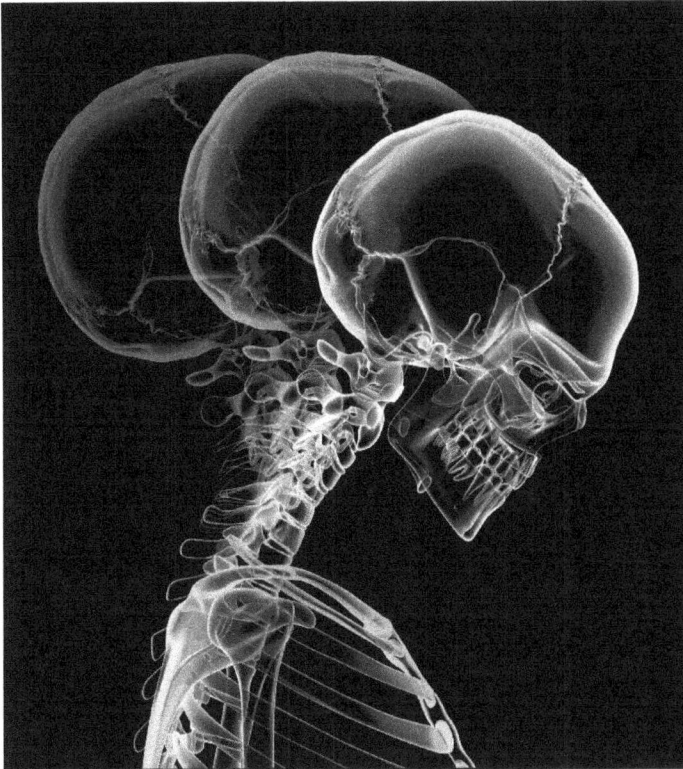

An overview of why you may hurt all over and what symptoms to watch out for after physical trauma.

By
DR. KARIN DRUMMOND, D.C.

—

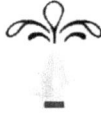

Published by Blooming Ink Publishing, LLC

4712 East State Road 46
Bloomington, IN 47401

FIRST EDITION

ISBN: 978-1-943753-09-3

Library of Congress Number: 2016913548

This book is dedicated to my patients and anyone who benefits from reading my books.

A special thank you to:

My husband, for being awesome at everything
 (Especially at adjusting spines).
My prolific and published daughter
 (Who infected me with the writer's bug).
My son, for being gentle with me when I was hurt.
Fine Art Images by George, LLC, for my image on the back cover.
Kip May Photography for my profile image.
Josh Gonzalez with EarWig Design for designing my book covers.
Vicki Adang, my professional editor, for taking on this project.
George Barnett for his contributions.
And countless others…

May this book be
my message in a bottle
in the sea of misinformation.

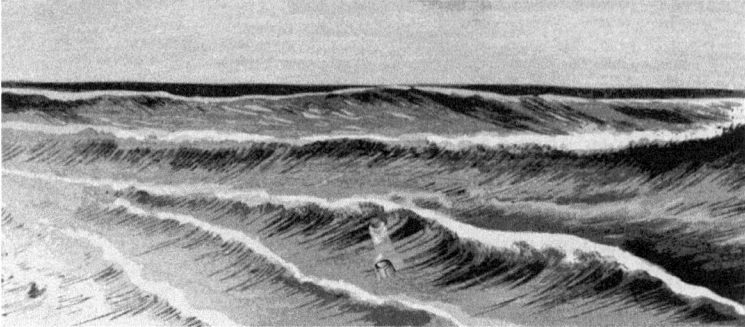

My mission is help you navigate through the labyrinth of
conflicting advice on how to live pain free and well.

Other books by Dr. Karin Drummond:
- **Top Seven Ways to Combat the Effects of Sitting**
- **Combat Slouching**
- **Combat Headaches**
- **Combat Irritable Bowels**
- **Whiplash to Wellness: A Chiropractor's Journey**

Up and coming books
- **Combat Jaw Pain**
- **Combat Neck Pain**
- **Combat Low Back Pain**
- **Combat Foot Pain**
- and many more…

Preface

Dear Reader,

I personally suffered with whiplash. I was shocked at how painful it was and mortified by how long it took me to recover. At the time of my accident, I had treated whiplash for fourteen years, and I thought I understood what it was and how to resolve it. My long journey of healing inspired me to write *Whiplash to Wellness: A Chiropractor's Journey* because if an expert struggled, I couldn't imagine how most whiplash sufferers faired. This book is just a sample of *Whiplash to Wellness,* which covers my experience and the lessons I learned in greater detail.

Having now experienced whiplash firsthand, I not only have a greater understanding of whiplash but a great deal more sympathy and newfound empathy for those suffering from it. On top of all that, now I have a true understanding of the legal aspects of whiplash.

I hope this book encourages you to read my all-inclusive *Whiplash to Wellness: A Chiropractor's Journey.* It explains why whiplash hurts so much and what such impact can do to the body (more than just neck pain), but more important, it explains what you can do about it. I am currently writing *Combat Neck Pain, Combat Low Back Pain* and *Combat Foot Pain* to explain in more detail what you can do if you suffer from these pains, whether or not yours is from an injury. I also plan on writing a book that will include answers to commonly asked legal questions about whiplash, as answered by my lawyer.

So many of my patients come in years after their accident with chronic pain they didn't know was likely due to an accident years earlier. If they had sought treatment earlier, they would have prevented arthritic changes later in life.

An ounce of prevention is worth a pound of cure!

Wishing you wellness,

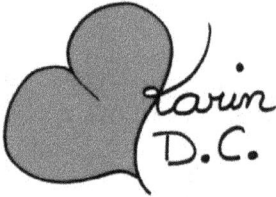

Karin Drummond, DC

TABLE OF CONTENTS:

Chapter 1: MY WHIPLASH STORY

As a chiropractor, I thought I understood whiplash pretty well. I had studied it and treated patients suffering from whiplash for over fourteen years at the time of my accident. But just like childbirth, you can't really understand it until you experience it yourself.

I experienced a severe case of whiplash after an accident in 2014. I thought the accident would just cause a mild case of whiplash, especially because I was super fit and healthy.

The Accident

I was driving straight through an intersection in good weather with nothing in front of me when, suddenly, a vehicle came out of nowhere and crossed the road right in front of me. My instincts took over, and I slammed on the brakes, despite having no time to stop. I T-boned her hard (Figure 1-1).

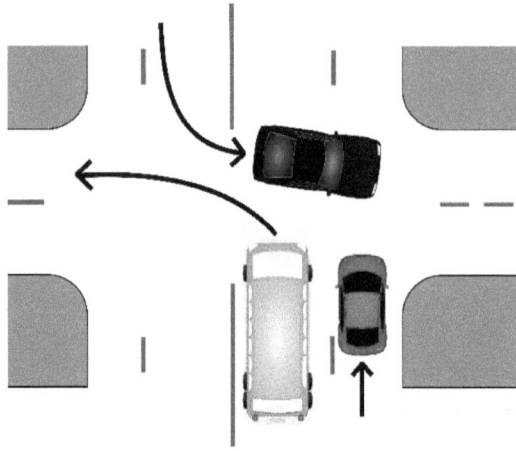

Figure 1-1: My small car T-boned the black SUV as it turned in front of me.

I was going at least 40 mph at the time of impact. My little Toyota Corolla hit the other driver's Jeep Cherokee so hard that it spun the SUV more than 180 degrees (Figure 1-2), and her back tire on the driver's side blew out when it hit the curb.

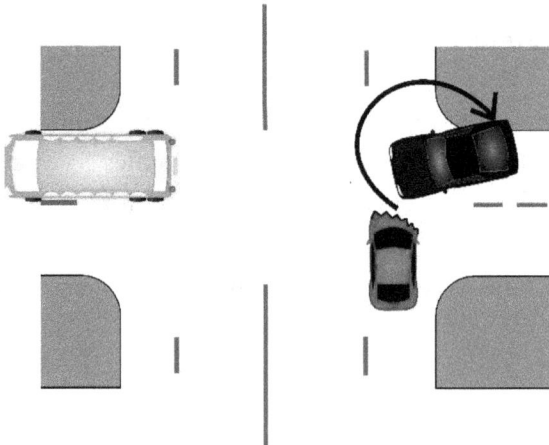

Figure 1-2: The black SUV spun 180 degrees after the impact.

With my body's forward momentum and my car going from

40 mph to zero in less than a second, my buttocks left the seat. My seat belt pressed hard against my chest, stopping me from hitting the steering wheel. I continued to brace, gripping the steering wheel intensely, expecting the airbag to deploy. I slammed back into my seat.

Note: Tensing was the kicker. I explain why tensing made my whiplash so much worse in *Whiplash to Wellness: A Chiropractor's Journey.*

My first thought was, *I must not have hit her as hard as I thought I would, or else the airbag would have deployed.*

I was dazed but didn't feel hurt. I closed my eyes and did a quick assessment. No bones felt broken. I could move all of my joints without pain. I opened my eyes. I didn't even see any cuts or bruises.

When I got out and looked at the damage to my car, I just thought I would be sore in the morning. I wasn't too worried. I was a tough cookie and married to a great chiropractor. I would be fine within a couple months, as healthy as I was.

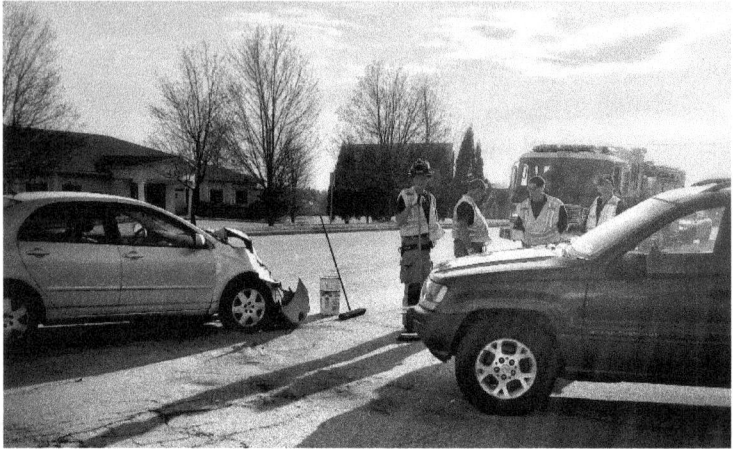

Figure 1-3: My car after the impact with the SUV

Boy, was I wrong. I had constant severe pain for weeks and on and off for months. It took me more than a year and a half to feel like I was strong and well again. Even today, I still have some vulnerabilities (no more headstands or roller coasters for me).

I write about my experience of recovering from whiplash in *Whiplash to Wellness: A Chiropractor's Journey*. I also plan to write a book with my attorney that explains how to pursue your legal claims. In spite of my initial reluctance to have an attorney help me, when it became clear that the other driver's insurance company didn't want to treat me fairly, I was glad I hired my lawyer.

For now, I will just say that you are entitled to have your medical and other expenses paid as well as receive compensation for the substantial pain and related difficulties you will likely experience during your recovery. And I can tell you firsthand that these are very real and the pain can be extremely debilitating.

Chapter 2: WHAT IS WHIPLASH?

Classically, whiplash is injury to the neck caused by a severe jerk to the body. The sudden movement, usually from a high-impact motor vehicle accident, causes the head to whip back and forth.

Every individual has different responses to whiplash. Every accident involves different forces from different vehicles in different environmental conditions. All of these variables make scientifically studying the effects of motor vehicle accidents on people difficult.

With this said, plenty of accidents occur daily, each one a learning experience. I was in a car accident that caused whiplash, so I am writing with not only firsthand knowledge of the pain and healing process but with now more than sixteen years as a chiropractor treating whiplash sufferers.

As an expert, I can say,

Whiplash is so much more than just neck pain!

Accidents that cause whiplash often also cause injuries to other parts of the body besides the neck and spine (Figure 2-1), including

- Feet
- Ankles
- Knees
- Hips
- Pelvis
- Wrists
- Elbows
- Shoulders
- Head
- Jaw
- Internal Organs

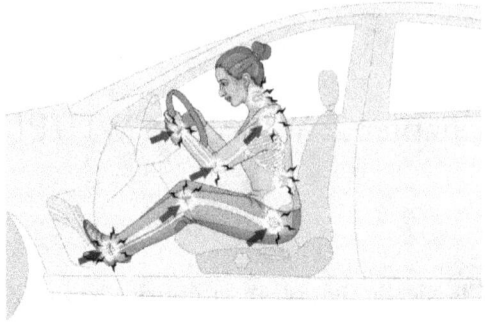

Figure 2-1: Forces affect more than just the neck.

You may not feel pain in these areas immediately after your accident, but don't be surprised if one day you experience pain with no apparent cause. I explain in Chapter 3 why it may take hours, days, or weeks to experience pain after an accident.

Chapter 3: YOU MAY BE INJURED EVEN THOUGH YOU'RE NOT IN PAIN

OFTENTIMES, PEOPLE HAVE NO PAIN after they've been in a car accident, so they think they are OK. Even I was guilty of this. But after a trauma, the mind and body go into some level of shock, minimizing the pain you feel, which clouds your judgment.

SEEK MEDICAL ATTENTION IMMEDIATELY AFTER AN ACCIDENT!

If Injury Occurs at the Time of the Accident, Why Don't I Feel Any Pain Right Away?

When our bodies experience pain or trauma, our "fight or flight" system kicks in. In prehistoric times, it was an advantage not to feel pain immediately. In those days when cavemen were injured, they couldn't afford to feel pain while the threat was still present. If they felt pain, they wouldn't be able to fight or flee from the cause of the injury; then they would likely die and not pass on their genes.

We still experience the "fight or flight" reaction today. When we are severely injured, our brains release beta-endorphins, which are basically powerful opiates that block pain.

After an accident, the damage is there; you just can't feel it. But over time, our kidneys filter these opiates out of our system, and we start to feel the effect of our injuries. Some people report pain three or four hours after the trauma; their injuries are so bad, they feel the pain as soon as the opiate levels start falling because it takes more opiates to block such severe pain. Other people may not feel any effects of the accident until the next day because it takes longer for the body to filter out the opiates to a level low enough to feel the pain.

If the pain starts two or more days after the trauma, then the person's pain is likely due to their compensation mechanisms causing injury. For example, a driver feels right knee pain weeks after the accident. This pain may be due to the arch of the right foot having dropped from the impact of slamming on the brakes during the accident. This can cause knee pain weeks later because the body has changed its gait cycle to compensate for the collapse of the right arch with every step. This altered gait places stress on the knee, slowly injuring it over time.

The moral of this story:
Seek medical attention after a car accident!

I can't stress this enough:
If you feel any pain,
GO TO THE EMERGENCY ROOM!

If you go to the ER and they say you are fine and give you

muscle relaxers and/or pain pills,

SEE A CHIROPRACTOR!

If you feel absolutely fine and decide not to go to the ER, at a minimum,

SEE A CHIROPRACTOR!

In my biased opinion, chiropractors are the most qualified to determine the level of your injuries. They are spine and joint experts. Medical doctors are disease experts. When it comes to spinal injuries, traditional medical doctors will prescribe pain pills, muscle relaxers, and if you are lucky, some physical therapy. Chiropractic offers so much more!

Knowing When to Talk to an Attorney

I asked my lawyer, George Barnett, how soon someone should contact a lawyer after suffering a whiplash injury. Here's his suggestion:

"While you generally have two years to file a lawsuit, it's a good idea to find and meet with a good lawyer as soon as possible after the accident. Your lawyer can assist you in gathering important evidence and advise you about making statements that may impact your claim. I always tell my clients to do everything they can to get better as soon as possible since nothing is worse then the ongoing pain. Holding out for money versus getting better is never an option. I can usually recommend very good people in the medical and chiropractic fields to assist them, and chiropractic treatment is often the most important contribution to recovery from whiplash injuries."

Chapter 4: EXPLAINING THE SEVERITY OF PAIN

WHEN I WAS AT MY WORST, I wondered how someone like me, who is strong, in shape, and flexible, could be in so much pain without having any scratches, bruises, or fractures, especially when I had no pain at the time of the accident!?!

Why Does it Hurt so Bad?

It makes sense that a broken bone hurts. You see a hard structure with a break in it. You see the cast that needs to be worn. For us visual creatures, it makes sense that a fractured bones hurts—a lot—and hurts as soon as it is broken.

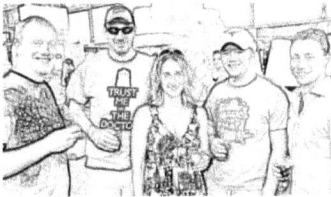

When I look at pictures of myself taken within two days of the accident, I can see why people didn't realize how hurt I was. You can't see how I couldn't move without searing pain because I wasn't moving. I simply couldn't turn my head because my protective muscles wouldn't let me. But just standing there, I looked great. So the pain couldn't be that bad, right?

A lawyer friend saw this picture on my Facebook page and advised me to stop posting pictures. He pointed out that the photos could be used against me in my personal injury case if it went to litigation, especially because it looked like I was fine and having fun.

My lawyer wasn't so concerned about that photo, but he pointed out that because injuries associated with whiplash are not as easy to see as a broken bone, the perception that nothing is really wrong or that people are faking the injury persists. Again, I know better. But I quit posting photos for a while anyway.

I can't state strongly enough how much pain I was in. There is just no way to describe the pain that does it justice. But why? Why is there so much pain in the neck and/or spine?

Before the advent of videography that could capture one thousand frames per second, the scientific explanation of whiplash was that the injury was simply due to the hyper-flexion/extension (head whipping back and forth) of the neck (Figure 4-1).

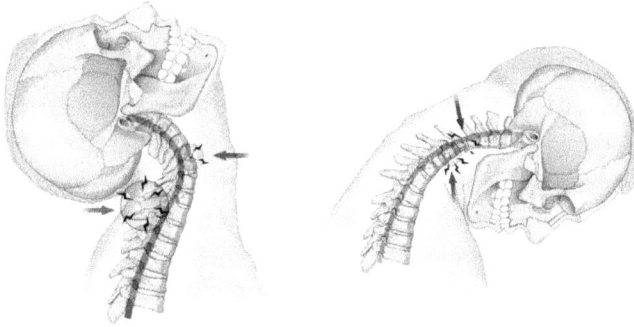

Figure 4-1: A hyper-flexion/extension injury.

Other experts would argue that the neck could handle such movement without injury, so whiplash was "faked" by people who were just looking to get more money out of their injury claims.

Since the late 1990s, with the ability to see what happens in the first 200 milliseconds of a deceleration injury, we have learned that damage occurs even before the head whips back and forth! At impact, damaging forces cause the vertebrae in the neck to slip forward in a very unnatural way (Figure 4-2).

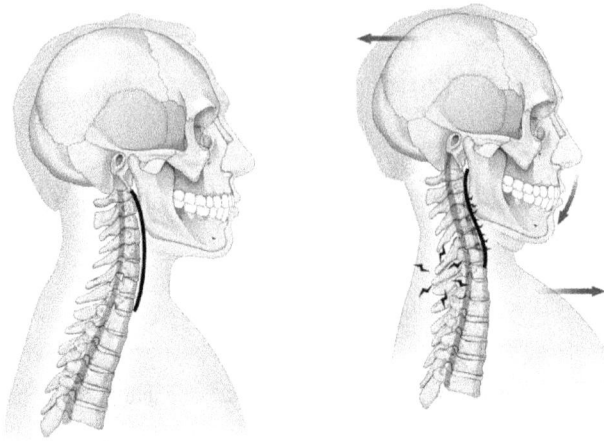

Figure 4-2: The dark lines depict the change of the curvature in the neck from a neutral C curvature to an aberrant S curvature in the first 200 milliseconds of impact.

This causes most of the damage. So much so, that when the head does whip back and forth, even further damage occurs!

Yes, a healthy, undamaged neck can handle a whipping back and forth action, but not after the damage sustained to the supporting ligaments of the neck that occurred in the first 200 milliseconds.

If you're curious about how whiplash injuries occur when you're hit from the back, front or side, you'll find more details in my *Whiplash to Wellness: A Chiropractor's Journey*.

What Speed Does It Take to Get Whiplash?

You can get whiplash at speeds much lower than those involved in a motor vehicle accident. I have had patients who have suffered from a whiplash injury after they've slipped on ice, jarring their body and causing their head to whip back in an unnatural position, resulting in further injury.

Why Do Low-Impact Collisions Hurt?

Whiplash is not a simple injury because not all bodies are the same. If you have a pre-existing but stable (asymptomatic) damaged region (like an old disc herniation) in your spine, you are more likely to experience pain after a whiplash injury than someone without these vulnerabilities. Or if you have experienced whiplash before, you are more likely to feel more pain than someone who has not.

People can have a wide variety of injuries with different levels of severity, even if they are in the same car!

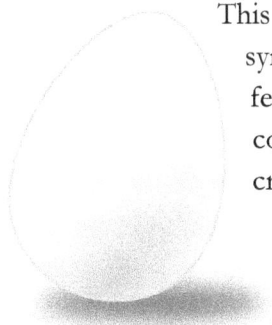

This has been called "the fragile egg syndrome," where a healthy egg feels fine after a high-impact collision, but a previously cracked egg was severely crippled by the same accident.

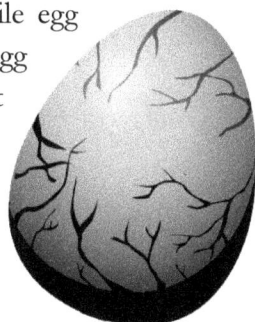

This is why it is so hard to predict how someone will do after any type of accident. Some people may need just a few treatments, while others may need a lifetime of care.

Remember, even if you feel fine after an accident, you may become a cracked "fragile egg" after an accident. This may make you more vulnerable to injury if you get involved in another accident. Please, even if you feel well, see a chiropractor (or at least some practitioner knowledgeable in whiplash injuries) who can help you mend your "silent" injuries.

If you do have pain in the neck, head, jaw, back, and/or foot pain, check out my other Combat Dis-ease books, like *Combat Headaches, Combat Jaw Pain,* etc.

Feel free to contact me at www.drummondchiropractic.com if you have a specific aliment that you would like for me to address in future publications.

I will continue to publish books to help those in pain or other states of dis-ease.

Chapter 5: MENTAL AND EMOTIONAL SYMPTOMS OF WHIPLASH

Whiplash can result in exhausting pain that seems like it will never end. Ongoing pain can affect the quality and quantity of sleep. Sleep deprivation alone can result in depression. Sleep deprivation compounded with searing pain that limits your ability to participate in your favorite activities—or even maintain your normal routine—can be overwhelmingly depressing. You may also find that you're more emotional for other reasons.

Severe Pain Can Result in Depression

Many people who experience whiplash ask themselves, their doctors, and others who have dealt with similar situations, "Am I ever going to get better?"

Even I, the eternally optimistic healer, succumbed to this question. I would tear up while wondering, "How is this going to affect my future if I can't do the things that keep me strong for my job?"

I nearly fell down the rabbit hole when I couldn't overcome my limitations and was too discouraged to even try. I almost let myself continue to weaken instead of focusing on how to strengthen. However, I realized I didn't want to live this way for the rest of my life, so I took steps to continue my recovery.

Severe Pain Can Amp Up Your Emotions

Severe pain married with sleep deprivation may make you more emotional. Add stress hormones to the mix, and you have the prime conditions for extreme emotional swings.

The best remedy is to let yourself cry. When you cry as a result of emotional stressors (extreme happiness or sadness), you release psychic tears. These tears can help you heal.

To learn how I coped with my depression and sudden emotional swings and how you can too, check out *Whiplash to Wellness: A Chiropractor's Journey.*

Chapter 6: BIOLOGICAL EFFECTS OF WHIPLASH

AFTER AN ACCIDENT, ask yourself every so often, "Am I experiencing any new complaints or symptoms since the accident?" No matter how unrelated the new symptoms may seem—for example, sneezing more often—they could be a result of injuries sustained during the accident.

Allergies and Your Immune System

Allergies occur when the body attacks pollen antigens thinking they are antigens on a virus or bacteria. This confusion leads to cold-like symptoms but without the actual sickness. When your body is confused, its defenses can hurt you instead of help you.

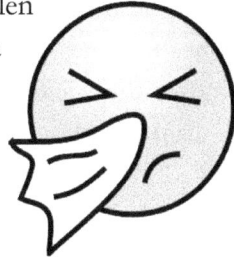

Physical trauma can also negatively affect your immune system. Your muscles may spasm, impinging on nerves that affect the immune system, causing it to malfunction.

Effect on Hormones

Your hormones may also change in response to increased

pain, sleep deprivation, and inflammation after an accident.

Over time, the stress of the pain can change the body's hormone levels, affecting your energy level, and cognitive function. Plus, fluctuating hormone levels can make you more sensitive to your pain, creating a vicious cycle.[1]

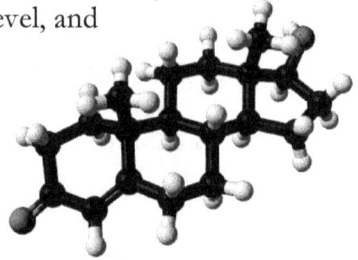

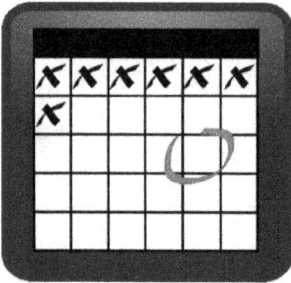

For women, hormone changes can affect their menstrual cycle. My first menses after my accident was a week early (I had never deviated more than a day since my last pregnancy seven years prior). The next one was a week late.

Some people experience lower thyroid levels months after whiplash injuries, leading to fatigue, weight gain, and other health issues. Because these symptoms often develop months after the accident, it can be difficult to trace their cause—a drop in thyroid levels—to the accident.

The moral of these examples,

Don't underestimate the effect of whiplash.

---

[1] University of Michigan Health System. "Pain and the Brain: Sex, Hormones & Genetics Affect Brain's Pain Control System." (February 18, 2003). www.eurekalert.org/pub_releases/2003-02/uomh-pat020703.php

Chapter 7: SYMPTOMS NOT TO IGNORE

RED-FLAG SYMPTOMS are those that require you to see a doctor immediately.

Seek immediate medical attention if (but not limited to)

- You have any numbness in the perineum, genitalia, and/or anus region (the area of your body that would touch the saddle if you were sitting in one). This can be a serious neurological condition called cauda equina syndrome. True numbness is when you cannot feel a thing.
  - o There are times when an area feels numb, but it's not completely numb. The feeling is duller (like there is cloth over your skin), but you can still feel someone pressing on your skin, just not as well. This is more of a paresthesia, which you shouldn't ignore. Have your doctor check it out.
- You have a loss of control of the bladder, genitalia, and/or bowels.
- You have muscle weakness where the muscles do not fire like your brain tells them to. For example, you try to walk and your foot does not lift up, or your grip is

weak

- You cannot find a position of relief. This can indicate an organ injury. In most musculoskeletal complaints, you can usually find a position that provides relief. If you are writhing around in pain, trying to find a comfortable position but can't, you likely have pain in an organ. If you are in a car accident and have abdominal pain that you cannot get relief from, it could be internal bleeding or organ damage.

- The pain is not going away after 4 to 6 weeks. In this case, the injury is not healing on its own, so seek professional advice.

- You have any changes in sight, taste, smell, personality, or memory, especially after a high-speed impact. These can be signs of a concussion or bleeding in the brain. You do not have to hit your head to injure your brain. Your brain can hit the inside of your skull and bruise.

- You are nauseous, pass out, or faint. These symptoms could be due to trauma to the heart or brain.

- You have difficulty swallowing. This can be the result of hemorrhaging in or tearing of the soft tissue in the front of the neck.

If you have any symptoms that concern you, contact one of your healing professionals for their opinion. It is always better to be safe than sorry. I have had many patients call me for my advice on symptoms they were concerned about. In the case of wellness, there truly is no stupid question because not asking can lead to serious and potentially irrevocable consequences.

With a basic understanding of whiplash and its potential consequences, you can begin putting together a team of healthcare providers to help you on your journey to wellness.

In my biased opinion, finding a qualified chiropractor is the first step. As with any profession, not all chiropractors are equal. Make sure the chiropractor you see has had success and plenty of experience with whiplash.

To discover your pathway to wellness, check out my book, *Whiplash to Wellness: A Chiropractor's Journey*, in which I not only share how to choose the best health care professionals for your specific needs, but I also reveal the treatments that helped me fully recover.

Let my story help you find your personal pathway from whiplash to wellness.

ABOUT THE AUTHOR

Karin Drummond, DC, lives in Bloomington, Indiana. She graduated with distinction from the University of Victoria with a bachelor of science degree. She finished the four-year doctorate of chiropractic degree at the University of Western States in 2000. She moved to her husband's hometown of Bloomington, Indiana, and has practiced there ever since. She now calls it home, living at its edge in the country with her husband and two children. She has been voted her town's number one chiropractor seven times as of 2016.

Passionate about living well, she keeps up with new research in the health field and practices what she preaches. Her patients have told her for years that she needed to write a book because she is such a great source of information on healthy living. Once she discovered how easy it was to publish a book, she decided to take advantage of this medium to help spread her thoughts on living well. Her first book, *Top Seven Ways to Combat the Effects of Sitting,* was published in 2015. She has published several books since then, and she is planning on publishing many more books on a variety of topics.

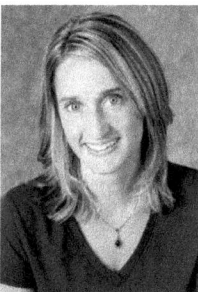

www.drummondchiropractic.com

ABOUT MY LAWYER AND CONTRIBUTOR

George Barnett graduated from the Indiana University School of Law in Bloomington, Indiana, in 1980. He has represented injured parties involved in serious injury and death cases throughout the United States for more than thirty years. He travels regularly to meet with top healthcare experts around the country who regularly assist him with his cases.

His experiences have given him considerable insight into the nature and impact of injuries across the spectrum, including soft tissue, whiplash, and brain injuries. George is passionate about seeking the best results for his clients' recoveries, and his compassion and his understanding of his clients' injuries is at the forefront of his representation. George has offices in Evansville and Bloomington, Indiana, and Boulder, Colorado.

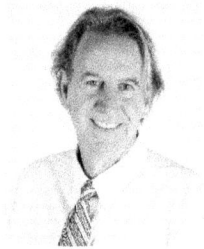

www.barnettinjurylaw.com.

Note from Dr. Karin: I was going to handle my case without a lawyer, and did for months. I was glad and relieved when I finally brought George onboard as my lawyer and supporter.

Other Books by Dr. Karin Drummond

Available now:

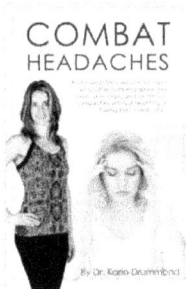

Combat Headaches
A chiropractor's advice for those who suffer from migraines, jaw pain, sinus pain, and/or tension headaches without resorting to taking pain medication.

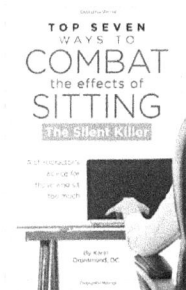

Top Seven Ways to Combat the Effects of Sitting: The Silent Killer
A chiropractor's advice for those who sit too much.

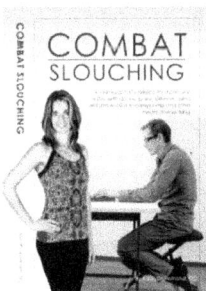

Combat Slouching
A chiropractor's advice for those who suffer from aches, pains, stiffness, spinal deformities, and other effects of slouching.

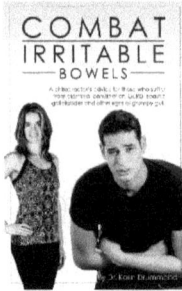

Combat Irritable Bowels

A chiropractor's advice for those who suffer from diarrhea, constipation, GERD, spastic gallbladder, and other signs of grumpy gut.

Coming soon:

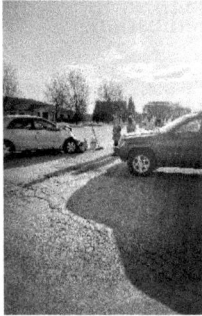

Whiplash to Wellness:
A Chiropractor's Journey

This is my personal journey that I am sharing to help others suffering from whiplash. This is my complete version that explains whiplash, and how to get well.

Up and Coming:
- **Combat Jaw Pain**
- **Combat Neck Pain**
- **Combat Low Back Pain**
- **Combat Foot Pain**
- and many other books…

All to help you find your personal path to wellness.

To find out more, visit Dr. Karin's website
www.drummondchiropractic.com

www.ingramcontent.com/pod-product-compliance
Lightning Source LLC
Chambersburg PA
CBHW060703280326
41933CB00012B/2287